THIS JOURNAL BELONGS TO:

_____

Goal Setting

As you start this journey it is important to make note of where you are today + where you want to go.

Setting goals is one of the best ways for you to hold yourself accountable + create success. In order to set strong goals you will want to track, reflect and evaluate your journey starting from day 1.

Use the next page to write specific goals that are based on what you measure for success. Below are some examples.

- Fitness Stats: running distance or speed, number of workout days per week, or one rep max.
- Lifestyle Goals: amount of sleep per night, reading or meditation.
- Nutritional Goals: water intake, trying new foods or cooking new recipes.
- Body Stats: weight, body fat percentage, or girth measurements.

Follow us on Instagram @PureFitnessWI for workouts, tips + accountability. Good Luck!

- Chellie, Annie + Jane -

My Goals

Self care is how you take your power back.

today's intention

date _____

positive affirmation

must get done today

1. _____ ☐
2. _____ ☐
3. _____ ☐

water intake

health + fitness

breakfast

lunch

dinner

snacks

today's intention

date _____

positive affirmation

must get done today

1. _____
2. _____
3. _____

water intake

health + fitness

breakfast

lunch

dinner

snacks

today's intention

date _____

positive affirmation

must get done today

1. _____

2. _____

3. _____

water intake

health + fitness

breakfast

lunch

dinner

snacks

today's intention

date _____

must get done today

1. _____ ☐

2. _____ ☐

3. _____ ☐

water intake

health + fitness

breakfast

lunch

dinner

snacks

today's intention

date _____

positive affirmation

must get done today

1. _____ ▢

2. _____ ▢

3. _____ ▢

water intake

health + fitness

breakfast

lunch

dinner

snacks

today's intention

date _____

positive affirmation

must get done today

1. _____ ☐

2. _____ ☐

3. _____ ☐

water intake

health + fitness

breakfast

lunch

dinner

snacks

today's intention

date _____

positive affirmation

must get done today

1. _____

2. _____

3. _____

water intake

health + fitness

breakfast

lunch

dinner

snacks

notes + doodles

date _____

today's intention

positive affirmation

must get done today

1. _____
2. _____
3. _____

water intake

health + fitness

breakfast

lunch

dinner

snacks

today's intention

date _____

positive affirmation

must get done today

1. _____ ☐

2. _____ ☐

3. _____ ☐

water intake

health + fitness

breakfast

lunch

dinner

snacks

today's intention

date _____

positive affirmation

must get done today

1. _____

2. _____

3. _____

water intake

health + fitness

breakfast

lunch

dinner

snacks

today's intention

date _____

positive affirmation

must get done today

1. _____

2. _____

3. _____

water intake

health + fitness

breakfast

lunch

dinner

snacks

date _____

positive affirmation

must get done today

1. _____ ☐

2. _____ ☐

3. _____ ☐

water intake

health + fitness

breakfast

lunch

dinner

snacks

date _____

today's intention

positive affirmation

must get done today

1. _____ ☐

2. _____ ☐

3. _____ ☐

water intake

💧 💧 💧 💧

💧 💧 💧 💧

health + fitness

breakfast

lunch

dinner

snacks

today's intention

date _____

positive affirmation

must get done today

1. _____

2. _____

3. _____

water intake

health + fitness

breakfast

lunch

dinner

snacks

notes + doodles

today's intention

date _____

positive affirmation

must get done today

1. _____ ☐

2. _____ ☐

3. _____ ☐

water intake

health + fitness

breakfast

lunch

dinner

snacks

today's intention

date _____

positive affirmation

must get done today

1. _____

2. _____

3. _____

water intake

health + fitness

breakfast

lunch

dinner

snacks

today's intention

date _____

positive affirmation

must get done today

1. _____

2. _____

3. _____

water intake

health + fitness

breakfast

lunch

dinner

snacks

today's intention

date _____

positive affirmation

must get done today

1. _____ ▢

2. _____ ▢

3. _____ ▢

water intake

health + fitness

breakfast

lunch

dinner

snacks

today's intention

date _____

positive affirmation

must get done today

1. _____

2. _____

3. _____

water intake

health + fitness

breakfast

lunch

dinner

snacks

today's intention

date _____

positive affirmation

must get done today

1. _____ ☐

2. _____ ☐

3. _____ ☐

water intake

health + fitness

breakfast

lunch

dinner

snacks

today's intention

date _____

positive affirmation

must get done today

1. _____
2. _____
3. _____

water intake

health + fitness

breakfast

lunch

dinner

snacks

today's intention

date _____

positive affirmation

must get done today

1. _____
2. _____
3. _____

water intake

health + fitness

breakfast

lunch

dinner

snacks

today's intention

date _____

positive affirmation

must get done today

1. _____
2. _____
3. _____

water intake

health + fitness

breakfast

lunch

dinner

snacks

today's intention

date _____

positive affirmation

must get done today

1. _____
2. _____
3. _____

water intake

health + fitness

breakfast

lunch

dinner

snacks

today's intention

date _____

positive affirmation

must get done today

1. _____

2. _____

3. _____

water intake

health + fitness

breakfast

lunch

dinner

snacks

today's intention

date _____

positive affirmation

must get done today

1. _____ ☐

2. _____ ☐

3. _____ ☐

water intake

health + fitness

breakfast

lunch

dinner

snacks

today's intention

date _____

positive affirmation

must get done today

1. _____

2. _____

3. _____

water intake

health + fitness

breakfast

lunch

dinner

snacks

WWW.PUREFITNESSWI.COM

today's intention

date _____

positive affirmation

must get done today

1. _____ ☐

2. _____ ☐

3. _____ ☐

water intake

health + fitness

breakfast

lunch

dinner

snacks

today's intention

date _____

positive affirmation

must get done today

1. _____

2. _____

3. _____

water intake

health + fitness

breakfast

lunch

dinner

snacks

today's intention

date _____

positive affirmation

must get done today

1. _____

2. _____

3. _____

water intake

health + fitness

breakfast

lunch

dinner

snacks

today's intention

date _____

positive affirmation

must get done today

1. _____

2. _____

3. _____

water intake

health + fitness

breakfast

lunch

dinner

snacks

today's intention

date _____

positive affirmation

must get done today

1. _____
2. _____
3. _____

water intake

health + fitness

breakfast

lunch

dinner

snacks

today's intention

date _____

positive affirmation

must get done today

1. _____
2. _____
3. _____

water intake

health + fitness

breakfast

lunch

dinner

snacks

today's intention

date _____

must get done today

1. _____ ☐

2. _____ ☐

3. _____ ☐

water intake

health + fitness

breakfast

lunch

dinner

snacks

today's intention

date _____

positive affirmation

must get done today

1. _____
2. _____
3. _____

water intake

health + fitness

breakfast

lunch

dinner

snacks

notes + doodles

today's intention

date _____

positive affirmation

must get done today

1. _____ ☐

2. _____ ☐

3. _____ ☐

water intake

💧 💧 💧 💧

💧 💧 💧 💧

health + fitness

breakfast

lunch

dinner

snacks

today's intention

date _____

positive affirmation

must get done today

1. _____ ☐

2. _____ ☐

3. _____ ☐

water intake

health + fitness

breakfast

lunch

dinner

snacks

today's intention

date _____

positive affirmation

must get done today

1. _____
2. _____
3. _____

water intake

health + fitness

breakfast

lunch

dinner

snacks

today's intention

date _____

positive affirmation

must get done today

1. _____

2. _____

3. _____

water intake

health + fitness

breakfast

lunch

dinner

snacks

today's intention

date _____

positive affirmation

must get done today

1. _____ ☐
2. _____ ☐
3. _____ ☐

water intake

💧 💧 💧 💧
💧 💧 💧 💧

health + fitness

breakfast

lunch

dinner

snacks

today's intention

date _____

positive affirmation

must get done today

1. _____ ☐

2. _____ ☐

3. _____ ☐

water intake

health + fitness

breakfast

lunch

dinner

snacks

today's intention

date _____

positive affirmation

must get done today

1. _____
2. _____
3. _____

water intake

health + fitness

breakfast

lunch

dinner

snacks

notes + doodles

today's intention

date _____

positive affirmation

must get done today

1. _____
2. _____
3. _____

water intake

health + fitness

breakfast

lunch

dinner

snacks

today's intention

date _____

positive affirmation

must get done today

1. _____ ☐

2. _____ ☐

3. _____ ☐

water intake

health + fitness

breakfast

lunch

dinner

snacks

today's intention

date _____

positive affirmation

must get done today

1. _____ ☐

2. _____ ☐

3. _____ ☐

water intake

health + fitness

breakfast

lunch

dinner

snacks

today's intention

date _____

must get done today

1. _____ ▢

2. _____ ▢

3. _____ ▢

water intake

💧 💧 💧 💧

💧 💧 💧 💧

health + fitness

breakfast

lunch

dinner

snacks

today's intention

date _____

positive affirmation

must get done today

1. _____ ☐

2. _____ ☐

3. _____ ☐

water intake

health + fitness

breakfast

lunch

dinner

snacks

today's intention

date _____

positive affirmation

must get done today

1. _____ ☐

2. _____ ☐

3. _____ ☐

water intake

💧 💧 💧 💧

💧 💧 💧 💧

health + fitness

breakfast

lunch

dinner

snacks

today's intention

date _____

positive affirmation

must get done today

1. _____ ☐

2. _____ ☐

3. _____ ☐

water intake

health + fitness

breakfast

lunch

dinner

snacks

notes + doodles

today's intention

date _____

positive affirmation

must get done today

1. _____

2. _____

3. _____

water intake

health + fitness

breakfast

lunch

dinner

snacks

today's intention

date _____

positive affirmation

must get done today

1. _____ ☐

2. _____ ☐

3. _____ ☐

water intake

health + fitness

breakfast

lunch

dinner

snacks

today's intention

date _____

positive affirmation

must get done today

1. _____
2. _____
3. _____

water intake

health + fitness

breakfast

lunch

dinner

snacks

today's intention

date _____

positive affirmation

must get done today

1. _____

2. _____

3. _____

water intake

health + fitness

breakfast

lunch

dinner

snacks

today's intention

date _____

positive affirmation

must get done today

1. _____

2. _____

3. _____

water intake

health + fitness

breakfast

lunch

dinner

snacks

today's intention

date _____

positive affirmation

must get done today

1. _____
2. _____
3. _____

water intake

health + fitness

breakfast

lunch

dinner

snacks

today's intention

date _____

positive affirmation

must get done today

1. _____ ▢

2. _____ ▢

3. _____ ▢

water intake

💧 💧 💧 💧

💧 💧 💧 💧

health + fitness

breakfast

lunch

dinner

snacks

notes + doodles

today's intention

date _____

positive affirmation

must get done today

1. _____
2. _____
3. _____

water intake

health + fitness

breakfast

lunch

dinner

snacks

today's intention

date _____

positive affirmation

must get done today

1. _____

2. _____

3. _____

water intake

health + fitness

breakfast

lunch

dinner

snacks

today's intention

date _____

positive affirmation

must get done today

1. _____ ☐

2. _____ ☐

3. _____ ☐

water intake

health + fitness

breakfast

lunch

dinner

snacks

date _____

today's intention

positive affirmation

must get done today

1. _____ ☐

2. _____ ☐

3. _____ ☐

water intake

💧 💧 💧 💧

💧 💧 💧 💧

health + fitness

breakfast

lunch

dinner

snacks

today's intention

date _____

positive affirmation

must get done today

1. _____
2. _____
3. _____

water intake

health + fitness

breakfast

lunch

dinner

snacks

today's intention

date _____

positive affirmation

must get done today

1. _____

2. _____

3. _____

water intake

health + fitness

breakfast

lunch

dinner

snacks

WWW.PUREFITNESSWI.COM

today's intention

date _____

positive affirmation

must get done today

1. _____

2. _____

3. _____

water intake

health + fitness

breakfast

lunch

dinner

snacks

notes + doodles

date _____

today's intention

positive affirmation

must get done today

1. _____

2. _____

3. _____

water intake

health + fitness

breakfast

lunch

dinner

snacks

today's intention

date _____

positive affirmation

must get done today

1. _____
2. _____
3. _____

water intake

health + fitness

breakfast

lunch

dinner

snacks

today's intention

date _____

positive affirmation

must get done today

1. _____ ☐

2. _____ ☐

3. _____ ☐

water intake

health + fitness

breakfast

lunch

dinner

snacks

today's intention

date _____

positive affirmation

must get done today

1. _____ ☐

2. _____ ☐

3. _____ ☐

water intake

health + fitness

breakfast

lunch

dinner

snacks

today's intention

date _____

positive affirmation

must get done today

1. _____ ☐

2. _____ ☐

3. _____ ☐

water intake

💧 💧 💧 💧

💧 💧 💧 💧

health + fitness

breakfast

lunch

dinner

snacks

today's intention

date _____

positive affirmation

must get done today

1. _____

2. _____

3. _____

water intake

health + fitness

breakfast

lunch

dinner

snacks

date _____

positive affirmation

must get done today

1. _____ ▢

2. _____ ▢

3. _____ ▢

water intake

💧 💧 💧 💧

💧 💧 💧 💧

health + fitness

breakfast

lunch

dinner

snacks

notes + doodles

today's intention

date _____

positive affirmation

must get done today

1. _____
2. _____
3. _____

water intake

health + fitness

breakfast

lunch

dinner

snacks

today's intention

date _____

positive affirmation

must get done today

1. _____ ☐

2. _____ ☐

3. _____ ☐

water intake

health + fitness

breakfast

lunch

dinner

snacks

today's intention

date _____

positive affirmation

must get done today

1. _____
2. _____
3. _____

water intake

health + fitness

breakfast

lunch

dinner

snacks

today's intention

date _____

positive affirmation

must get done today

1. _____

2. _____

3. _____

water intake

health + fitness

breakfast

lunch

dinner

snacks

today's intention

date _____

positive affirmation

must get done today

1. _____ ☐

2. _____ ☐

3. _____ ☐

water intake

health + fitness

breakfast

lunch

dinner

snacks

today's intention

date _____

positive affirmation

must get done today

1. _____ ▢

2. _____ ▢

3. _____ ▢

water intake

health + fitness

breakfast

lunch

dinner

snacks

today's intention

date _____

positive affirmation

must get done today

1. _____ ☐

2. _____ ☐

3. _____ ☐

water intake

💧 💧 💧 💧

💧 💧 💧 💧

health + fitness

breakfast

lunch

dinner

snacks

WWW.PUREFITNESSWI.COM

notes + doodles

today's intention

date _____

positive affirmation

must get done today

1. _____
2. _____
3. _____

water intake

health + fitness

breakfast

lunch

dinner

snacks

today's intention

date _____

positive affirmation

must get done today

1. _____
2. _____
3. _____

water intake

health + fitness

breakfast

lunch

dinner

snacks

today's intention

date _____

positive affirmation

must get done today

1. _____
2. _____
3. _____

water intake

health + fitness

breakfast

lunch

dinner

snacks

today's intention

date _____

positive affirmation

must get done today

1. _____ ☐

2. _____ ☐

3. _____ ☐

water intake

health + fitness

breakfast

lunch

dinner

snacks

today's intention

date _____

positive affirmation

must get done today

1. _____ ☐

2. _____ ☐

3. _____ ☐

water intake

health + fitness

breakfast

lunch

dinner

snacks

today's intention

date _____

positive affirmation

must get done today

1. _____ ☐

2. _____ ☐

3. _____ ☐

water intake

health + fitness

breakfast

lunch

dinner

snacks

today's intention

date _____

positive affirmation

must get done today

1. _____
2. _____
3. _____

water intake

health + fitness

breakfast

lunch

dinner

snacks

Printed in Great Britain
by Amazon

19097762R00058